richa

HOW TO
REDUCE AND
SURVIVE CANCER

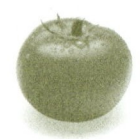

First published 2009

Copyright © 2009

Reprinted 2014.

All rights reserved. No part of this publication may be reproduced in any form without prior permission from the publishers.

British Library Cataloguing in Publication Data. A catalogue record for this book is available from the British Library.

ISBN 978-1-906381-59-2

Published by Autumn House, Grantham, Lincolnshire.
Printed in China.

In nature there are neither rewards nor punishments – there are consequences.
Robert E. Ingersoll

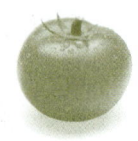

CANCER, kan'sər...

... loosely any malignant new growth or tumour: properly a carcinoma or disorderly growth of epithelial cells which invade adjacent tissue and spread by the lymphatics and blood vessels to other parts of the body.... [Latin, *crab.*]
Chamber's Twentieth Century Dictionary

Cancer is not a fate, it is a matter of risk, and you can adjust those risks by how you behave. It is very important that people feel that they are in control of what they do.
Professor Martin Wiseman

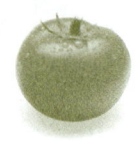

Cancer

- It is a word – not a sentence.
- It is also called *malignancy* or *neoplasia*, and is a disease of uncontrolled cell growth.
- Around 10 million billion cells in the human body co-operate over three score years and ten to keep us healthy.
- There are about 200+ types of cancer.
- It is not contagious and only a few are inherited.
- It will affect 1 in 3 persons over a lifetime.

... the incidence of cancer throughout the world can be reduced by 30 to 40% by feasible changes in diet and related lifestyles.
World Cancer Research Fund

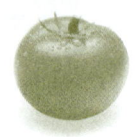

A European Communities Commission Report

showed that of cancer deaths:
- one third are attributed to diet, particularly alcohol;
- one third to cigarette smoking;
- one third to infection, sexual and reproduction behaviours and occupational activities.

Europe against cancer

Started in 1987, the aim is to reduce cancer mortality across 75 action areas by 15% through:
- fighting the tobacco habit
- nutrition
- protection against carcinogenic agents
- screening and early detection
- reduction of alcohol consumption
- improvement in gynaecological hygiene
- moderation in sun tanning

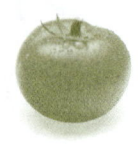

- About 40% of all cancers are beyond possible control.
- The ECC aims to reduce even this level to at most 10%.

How cancer arises

Traditional research has been in the following areas:
- Cancer is a genetic disease. Alterations to the DNA inside cells can endow cells with morbid 'super-powers', such as the ability to grow anywhere and to continue dividing indefinitely.
- Most cancer research has focused on mutations to a relatively small set of cancer-related genes as the decisive events in the transformation of healthy cells to malignant tumours.

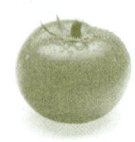

- New research centres on:
  1. a breakdown in DNA duplication or repair leading to many thousands of random mutations in cells.
  2. damage to a few 'master' genes mangles the chromosomes, which then become dangerous.
  3. abnormal numbers of chromosomes in a cell may be the first milestone on the road to cancer.

Four characteristics of cancer

1. Abnormal cells:
Anaplasia, where the cells do not differentiate and develop normally.

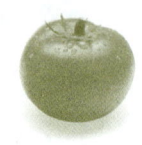

2. Cloning:

A cell undergoes particular genetic changes or mutations and then reproduces clones of its new form over and over again.

3. Metastasis:
The spread of cancer cells via the blood or lymphatic system to other sites in the body where they settle and grow.

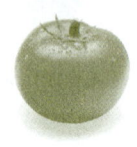

4. Unregulated growth:
Since the cell growth is unregulated it becomes excessive and under its own autonomous control.

Cell abnormalities
1. Growth without the proper signals for growth in which the cancer cells 'counterfeit' pro-growth messages to the cell.

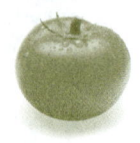

2. Over-riding stop signals in which the malignant cells ignore the chemical messages to stop cell growth and division.

3. Evading inherent auto-destruct mechanisms, in which the malignant cells bypass the system which would automatically destroy rogue cells.

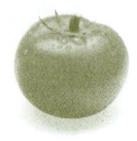

4. Co-opting nearby blood vessels to provide cell nutriment and oxygen to the growing mass.

5. Work around the *telomere* system at the *chromosome* edges to overcome the normal 70 times division rate to divide indefinitely.

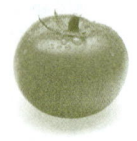

6. Interference with other vital tissues and organs, thus creating a life-threatening environment in the body.

Tumours
- Many cancers take the form of tumours, a new growth of body tissue having no purpose or contribution to make to the function of the body.
- Tumours may be *malignant* – they spread or *metastasise* to other parts of the body – or *benign* when they do not spread out of control.

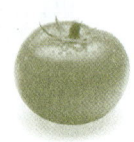

Just a sample

- A biopsy in which a small piece of the suspect tissue is removed for examination tests whether the tumour is malignant or benign.
- This can be done in the GP surgery, although some biopsies will require surgery.

Principal causes of cancer

Cause	Estimated percentage of all cancer deaths (%)
Tobacco	30
Alcohol	3
Diet	35
Food additives	Less than 1
Occupation	4
Pollution	2
Industrial products	Less than 1
Medicines and medical procedures	1
Infection	10
Other and unknown	13

R. Doll, R. Peto

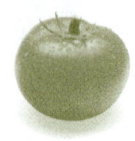

Top three causes of cancer death

Men
1 Lung cancer
2 Colon cancer
3 Prostate cancer

Women
Breast cancer
Colon cancer
Cancer of ovaries/uterus

Common cancer screening tests

- Self-examination of breasts and testicles.
- Rectal exams every year after age 40.
- Blood tests of stools every year after age 50.
- Cervical (PAP – *Papanicolaou*) smear test
  - within 6 months of first intercourse
  - 6-12 months later
  - approximately 3-year intervals thereafter.

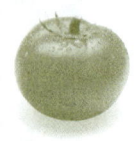

Common cancer sites
1. Brain tumour
- *Primary* (if arising in the skull), *secondary* (if spread from elsewhere)
- More common age 50+
- Cranial pressure, headache, vomiting, impairment of the senses, muscle weakness, and epileptic fits
- Surgical removal where possible and anti-cancer drugs enhance survivability.

2. Breast cancer
- Most common cancer in women worldwide
- Painless hard lump doubling in size every three months in the breast
- Lump may be a fluid-filled cyst, a thickening in the milk-producing tissue *(fibroadenoma)*, a benign tumour, breast cancer
- Surgical removal of the lump or the breast and a range of anti-cancer treatments will determine risks and survivability.

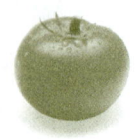

Strong associations for breast cancer risk include:
- early onset of menstruation
- increasing age
- a family history of breast cancer in a first-degree relative, i.e. mother
- having the first child when 30+
- no children
- late menopause
- the contraceptive pill
- obesity
- exposure to radiation

Weight and relative risk of female breast cancer

Weight	Pre-menopausal	Post-menopausal
Thin	1.00	1.00
Normal	1.29	4.76
Slightly obese	2.10	4.51
Obese	2.98	12.38

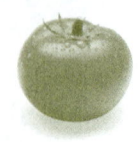

Breast cancer odds

20 years old   1:2,500
30 years old   1:233
40 years old   1:65
50 years old   1:41
60 years old   1:29
70 years old   1:24
80 years old   1:16
90 years old   1:8

Cancer and ethnicity

- African-Americans are 60% more likely to develop and twice as likely to die from prostate cancer as their white compatriots.
- Women of African-American descent have slightly less breast cancer than their counterparts but it strikes them at a younger age and is more lethal in its outcome.
- UK black women may develop breast cancer two decades before white women (average age 46 compared with 67 respectively).

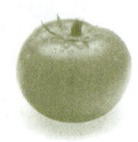

Some dietary associations in breast cancer risk

Study of 90,000 women aged 26-46:
- Daily consumption of red meat doubles the risk of breast cancer.
- Growth hormones given to cattle, or chemicals added during meat processing could fuel hormone-responsive cancers.
- Hormone-responsive cancers account for two-thirds of breast cancers.

Archives of Internal Medicine

Dr Hiruyamama in a study of meat and egg use in Japanese women with breast cancer showed:

Frequency of use	Meat	Eggs
Once a week	General	General
2-4 times a week	2.6	1.9
Daily	3.8	2.8

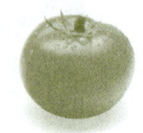

Fat consumption and breast cancer

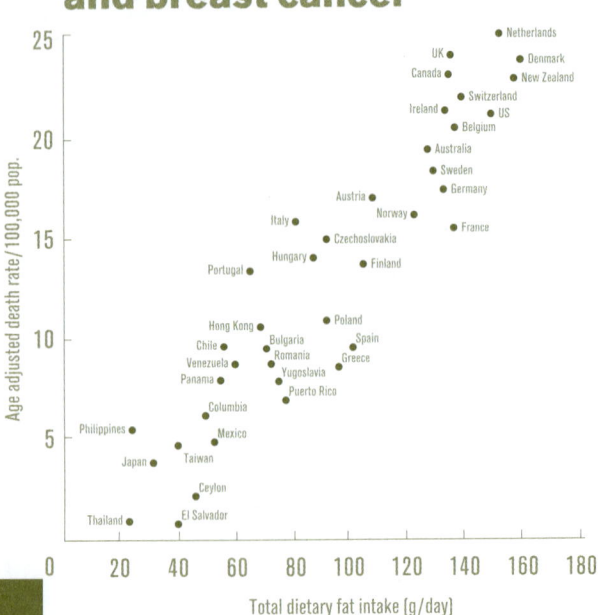

Fibre and breast cancer
- Pre-menopausal women who have the greatest intake of fibre decrease their risk of breast cancer by half.
British Journal of Cancer

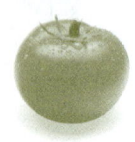

Alcohol and breast cancer

- One alcoholic drink a day raises breast cancer risk by 6%.
- At five alcoholic drinks a day there is 30% more risk than teetotallers of having breast cancer.

Exercise and breast cancer

- Women who take frequent exercise on a lifelong lifestyle basis may reduce the risk of breast cancer by 30%.

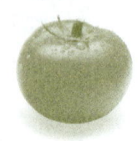

Keeping at it

A 2005 study showed that 92% of nearly 3,000 women with breast cancer who walked or did other exercise three to five hours weekly were still alive ten years after their diagnosis, compared with 86% of those who exercised less than an hour a week.
Scientific American

Breast self-examination

- Be aware of your breasts' general shape and size, and look each month for any change.
- Raising each arm in turn above your head, look from side to side for any changes in appearance.
- Check, by gently squeezing the nipples, for any discharge.

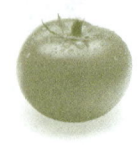

- Look at the skin surface and note any changes – an 'orange-peel' texture might indicate an underlying lump.
- Lie, supported by a pillow under the neck and shoulder, and use the flat of your hand in a clockwise direction, feeling around the outer part of the breast.
- With one arm raised above the head, use the flat of the other hand to examine the inner parts of the breast, top of the collarbone, and armpit. (Change pillow to opposite shoulder and repeat with the other breast.)

3. Cervical cancer
- Most prevalent in sexually-active young women exposed to the transmission of the *human papilloma virus* (HPV).
- Two types: *squamous cell, adenocarcinoma*.
- Can spread to other pelvic organs.
- Smear test will reveal abnormal changes *(dysplasias)* to the cervix and vaginal bleeding at unexpected times.

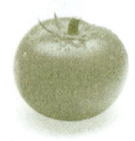

- Treatment may be by electrocoagulation, diathermy, laser treatment, cryosurgery (application of intense cold), radiotherapy, surgery, and/or a range of anti-cancer drugs.
- Survival rates: if early-detected, 50-80%; if later, 10-30%; or, with radical surgery, 30-50%.
- The treatment rates are highly successful if the cancer is limited only to the cervix.

HRT and cancer

- Combined HRT use doubles the risk of breast cancer.
- Postmenopausal women using HRT showed a 20% increased risk of developing and dying from ovarian cancer than non-users.
- Stopping HRT returned the ovarian cancer risk to normal within a few years.
- The total incidence of ovarian, breast and womb (endometrial) cancers is estimated to be 63% higher in HRT users.

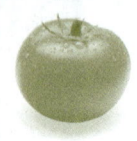

4. Colon cancer

- The second most common cancer for men and women worldwide with around 5% due to an inherited predisposition.
- Develops from colon polyps (new growths).
- Change in bowel habits and blood in the stools.
- May be lower abdominal pain or tenderness.
- Cancer confirmed by sigmoidoscopy.
- 70% of colon cancer may be prevented by a healthy lifestyle.

Bile acids and colon cancer

Individuals on a high-animal-fat diet (the Western diet) produce more bile acids, particularly *lithocholic* and *taurodeoxycholic*, which have been shown to enhance tumour growth. It has been observed that people with colon cancer produce more bile acids than people without colon cancer.

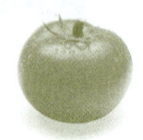

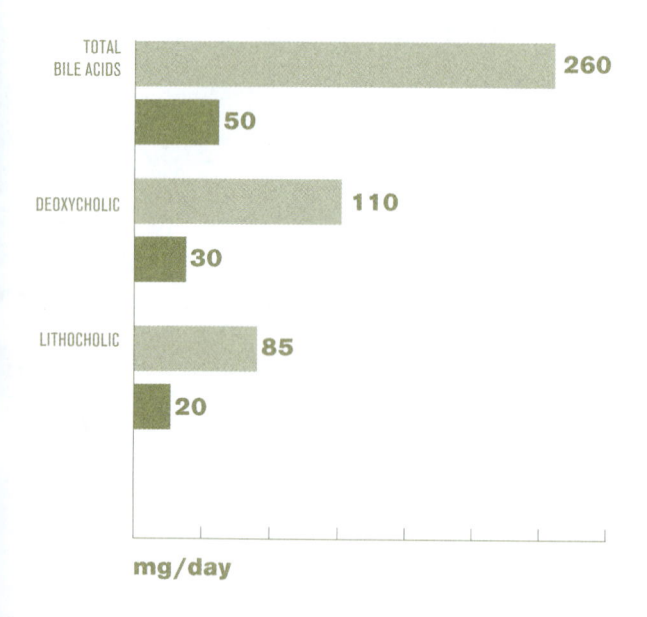

	mg/day
TOTAL BILE ACIDS	Americans: 260
	Seventh-day Adventists, Japanese, Chinese, American Vegetarians: 50
DEOXYCHOLIC	Americans: 110
	Seventh-day Adventists, Japanese, Chinese, American Vegetarians: 30
LITHOCHOLIC	Americans: 85
	Seventh-day Adventists, Japanese, Chinese, American Vegetarians: 20

Meat consumption and colon cancer

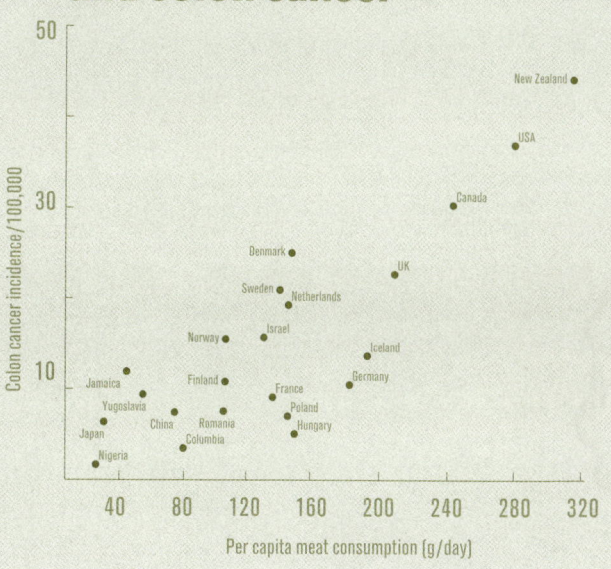

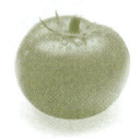

Possible relationship between diet and bowel cancer

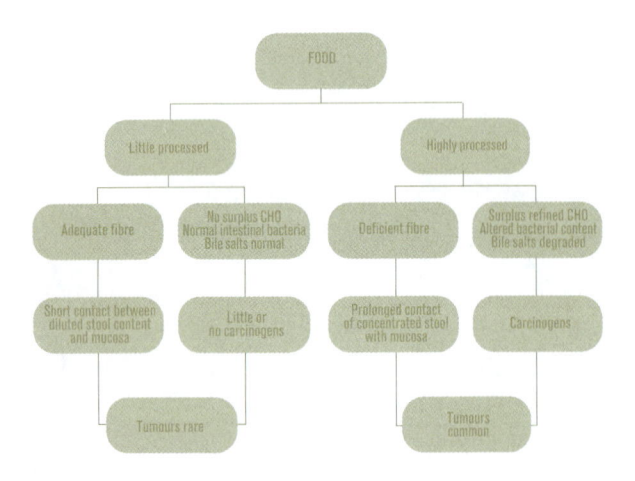

```
                          FOOD
                         /    \
              Little processed   Highly processed
                /    \              /    \
        Adequate    No surplus CHO    Deficient   Surplus refined CHO
        fibre       Normal intestinal bacteria   fibre       Altered bacterial content
                    Bile salts normal                         Bile salts degraded
          |              |                    |                    |
  Short contact between  Little or      Prolonged contact    Carcinogens
  diluted stool content  no carcinogens  of concentrated stool
  and mucosa                             with mucosa
            \            /                    \            /
             Tumours rare                      Tumours common
```

Top five countries with *the worst rates of stomach cancer*

- Belarus
- Russia
- Ukraine
- Estonia
- Croatia

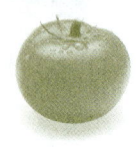

Salt and cancer
- A Japanese study showed the risk of stomach cancer was 1:500 a year for men with the highest salt intake (twice the rate of those using salt least).
- The risk in women was 1:1,300 compared to 1:2,000 for a relatively salt-free diet.

Exercise and bowel cancer
- Exercise of a regular and moderate intensity can halve the risk of developing bowel cancer.

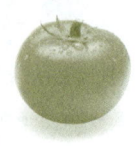

Diabetes and bowel cancer

People with diabetes could be up to three times more likely to get bowel cancer with the trend being stronger in men than in women.
Professor Kay-Tee Khaw

5. Leukaemia

- An either acute or chronic cancer of the white blood cells.
- Several different types.
- Characterised by anaemia, bleeding gums, easily bruised body, headache and bone tenderness.
- Confirmed by blood tests.
- Usually treated with chemotherapy and/or bone marrow transplant.
- Outlook for survival dependent on type of leukaemia.

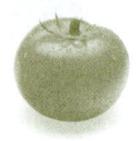

Vanity risk

- Women who use hair dyes more than 9 times a year have a 60% greater risk of *chronic lymphocytic leukaemia*, according to a Yale School of Public Health Report.

6. Liver cancer

- *Primary* (if originating in the liver) and of two types, *hepatoma* being the most common; *secondary* (if spread from elsewhere).
- Loss of weight, appetite, and energy.
- May be upper abdominal pain, jaundice and excess abdominal fluid.
- Primary cancer may be cured by removal of the tumour, or slowed by chemotherapy; while there is no cure for secondary cancer, progress may be slowed by drugs.

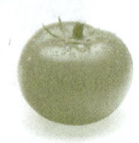

7. Lung cancer

- The number one cause of cancer death.
- Several types, of which *squamous cell, small* and *large cell* are related to cigarette use (in about 90% of males and 80% of females).
- Risk is 20 times higher for a pack-a-day smoker compared with a non-smoker; and a 30% risk of developing the cancer from passive smoking (living in the same household as the smoker).

- Typically characterised by a chronic cough (which may contain blood), chest pain, bronchitis, wheezing and shortness of breath.
- Treated by removal of all or part of the affected lung, anti-cancer drugs or radiotherapy.
- 15-30% survival rate after surgery.

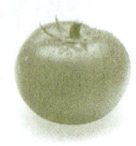

Exercise and lung cancer

- A study of 14,000 men 50+ showed that moderate regular exercise reduced the risk of lung cancer by 40%.

8. Lymphomas
- Two types: *Hodgkin's disease* (if abnormal Reed-Sternberg cells present), or *non-Hodgkin's lymphoma*.
- More common in age range 30-40 with the latter type mostly in people 50+.
- Affects mainly the lymph nodes and spleen which may be painless or enlarged, or pain and swelling in the lymph nodes of the neck or groin.
- High cure rate.

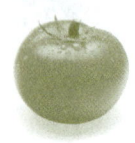

9. Ovarian cancer

- The third most common cancer in women (with *uteran* cancer).
- Typically occurring in the over-50s and not usually detected early.
- Accompanied by abdominal discomfort and swelling, nausea, vomiting and vaginal bleeding.
- Treated with anti-cancer drugs, surgery, radiotherapy.
- 60-70% survival of 5+ years.

10. Pancreatic cancer

- Has a poor prognosis as the cancer is fairly widespread when diagnosed.
- People with pancreatic cancer typically present with: painless jaundice, upper abdominal pain, loss of appetite and weight, nausea, diarrhoea, vomiting and tiredness.
- No high survival rate in advanced cases, but may be cured if detected early and treated with anti-cancer drugs.

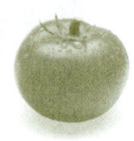

11. Prostate cancer

- The third most common cancer in men from middle-age.
- Enlargement of prostate with difficulty in passing urine.
- Maybe pain in bones from secondary cancer.
- Non-specific treatment if small; surgery or radiotherapy; and testosterone-blocking drugs.

- The average doubling time of prostate cancer (15 months) can be slowed by the anti-inflammatory effect of an 8oz/0.24 litre glass of pomegranate juice daily to 54 months.

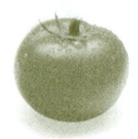

Fat consumption and prostate cancer

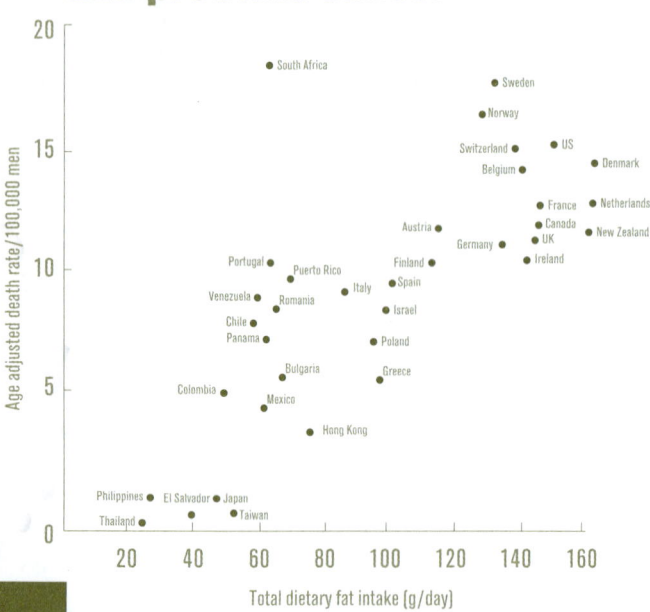

Omega oils

Eating a diet with the right balance of omega-3 and omega-6 fats may well help to keep prostate cancer within the prostate gland.
Noel Clarke

It is possible to have a healthy balance of these two types of fat – we only need about half as much omega-3 as omega-6 – that will stop cancer cells from spreading.
Dr Mick Brown

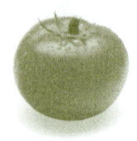

Cholesterol and prostate cancer

- High cholesterol levels, especially in the West, accelerate the growth of prostate tumours.
- Prostate cancers are up to 90% less in parts of rural China and Japan where the dietary cholesterol intake is low.

Vitamins and prostate cancer

- A journal of the National Cancer Institute (US) reported that taking multivitamins more than seven times a week may *increase* prostate cancer risk by up to 32%.

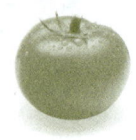

12. Skin cancer

- May be *basal cell*, *squamous cell*, or *melanoma*, only the latter of which is life-threatening.
- Length and intensity of exposure to ultraviolet light determines the risk; or exposure to other skin irritants.
- Prevented by sun-screen and appropriate clothing and other specific protective measures, depending on the cause.

- Is estimated to treble over the next 30 years, mainly due to overseas holidays and global warming.
- Rates of *malignant melanoma* are rising faster than any other type of cancer.
- The increased use of tanning equipment is a minor contributory factor.

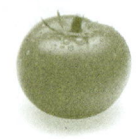

Moles and moles

Use the **ABCD** system to see if a mole is suspicious.

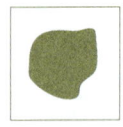

A is the *asymmetry* of the mole (normally round, but melanomas oddly shaped).

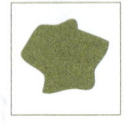

B is for *border* irregularity with malignant melanomas diffusing edge colour into surrounding skin.

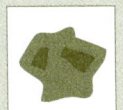

C variation in *colour* with a mixture of colours (mainly dark brown or black) raising the suspicion of a malignancy.

D the *diameter* of the mole (size in itself is not a diagnosis, but the mole's growth may be significant and generally a size of 6mm/¼ inch plus may be suspect).

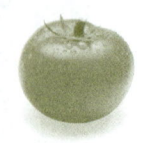

13. Throat (pharynx) cancer

- Usually associated with the use of tobacco smoking (past or present), smokeless tobacco, or alcohol, but many different causes and symptoms.
- It easily metastasises and has a poor cure rate.
- Typically difficulty in swallowing, or a lump in the throat.
- Survival depends on the site and type of cancer and the person's age.

HPV and cancer
- A study reported in *Cancer* found that *human papillomavirus* (HPV) infection is linked to a rise in tonsil and tongue cancers, particularly among men younger than 45.

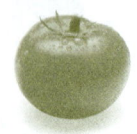

Survival

- To live beyond
- To outlive
- To remain alive

From Latin: *super* – beyond
 vivere – to live

Survival has different interpretations. To the

Cancer patient: Survival means people living at any period apparently free of recurrent or persistent cancer.
Oncologists: Survival begins from the time of diagnosis for statistical purposes, that is, living at time X.
Lay carers: Survival describes their own state of continued life beyond the death of the one for whom they cared.
Support groups: Survival refers to everyone living after a cancer diagnosis.

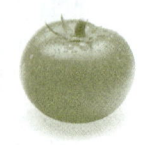

Five-year survival rates for various cancers (%)

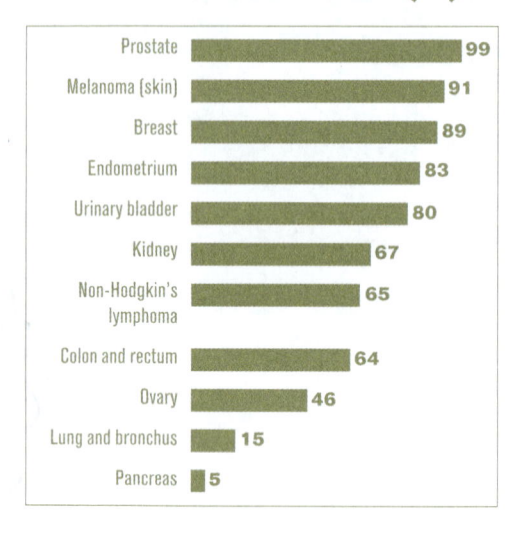

Prostate	99
Melanoma (skin)	91
Breast	89
Endometrium	83
Urinary bladder	80
Kidney	67
Non-Hodgkin's lymphoma	65
Colon and rectum	64
Ovary	46
Lung and bronchus	15
Pancreas	5

Breast cancer survival rate:
- Where the individual lacked social support = 18.9 months.
- Where support was available = 36.6 months.

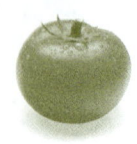

Positive thinking

... neither the state of the tumour nor the psychological state of the patient predicted how long he or she would live ... the severity of physical symptoms, such as nausea, weakness and difficulty in breathing, were the best indicators that life would soon come to an end.
Antonio Vigano et al, University Health Centre, Montreal

Too much bottle!
A 30-year review of the scientific literature, published in 2004, suggested that cancer patients who feel helpless or who suppress negative emotions may be at greater risk of having their cancer spread than those who play a role in their healing.
Scientific American

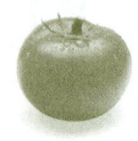

Duke University study of 1,718 men and women aged 65+

found an association between increased immune function and regular attendance at religious services.
International Journal of Psychiatry in Medicine

Survival rate over a 20-year period is better for the socially involved.

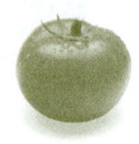

An individual's physical and mental health is profoundly affected by other people. Our health is in some way crucially dependent on other people, and we ourselves may be instrumental in affecting the health of others.

Cancer and cognition
- Cancer survivors may be at increased risk of problems with mental abilities such as those involving memory and learning.
- Cognitive problems are twice as likely to occur in people who have undergone cancer treatment.
- About 15% of cancer survivors have signs of cognitive dysfunction.

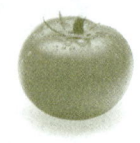

The public has the notion that fat gives you heart disease and diabetes, but they don't realise it also gives you cancer. . . . After smoking, obesity is the highest preventable cancer risk.
Professor Martin Wiseman

Cancers linked to obesity

Bowel
Breast
Kidney
Leukaemia
Multiple myeloma (bone marrow)
Non-Hodgkin's lymphoma
Oesophagus
Ovarian
Pancreatic
Womb

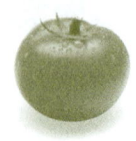

Cancer in general, and exercise

- Physical activity of a regular nature is thought to reduce the risks of endometrial, prostate and testicular cancers and may play a role in lowering cancer risk across a range of cancers.

Diet and cancer

It is our current estimate that some 50% of all female cancers in the Western world and about one third of all male cancers are related to nutritional factors.
Ernest Wynder, American Health Foundation

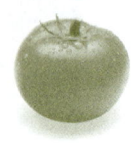

In the Framingham Study those men whose total cholesterol levels were below 190mg/dl were more than three times as likely to get colon cancer as those men with cholesterol greater than 220; they were almost twice as likely to contract any kind of cancer than those with cholesterol over 280mg/dl.
Gary Taubes

Blood sugar and cancer
- Swedish research showed a link with raised blood sugar levels and an increase in pancreatic, skin, womb and urinary tract cancers in women.
- For women under age 49, high blood sugar levels were linked to a higher incidence of breast cancer.

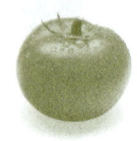

Oh, rats! Another reason to diet

Rodent studies have shown that
- eating your fill may promote cancer by boosting a harmful blood protein.
- *IGF-1* (Insulin-like Growth Factor-1) given to rats caused the development of multiple tumours.
- one third less calories increased the rat lifespan by 30%.

BBQs
- High temperature cooking methods, such as grilling, broiling and frying release *Advanced Glycation End Products* (AGEs) in meats and cheeses, which increase the risk of life-threatening diseases, such as heart disease, kidney disease, diabetes and brain damage.
JRSH

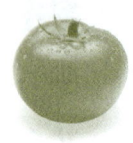

- Reducing the BBQ temperature will help to offset the effects.
- Keeping food moist during the cooking process will help to minimise the risk.
- Using mildly acidic marinades and condiments will also help to counteract the effect.

BBQs

Charcoal BBQs release:
Benzopyrene

A charcoal-broiled steak of 1kg/2.2lbs = cigarette smoke from 600 cigarettes.

Oral benzopyrene produces stomach tumours, leukaemia.

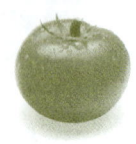

Dye, the death!
- Around 350 foods have been found to contain the dye Sudan I, normally used as a colouring agent in solvents, oils, waxes, petrol, and shoe and floor polishes, linked to an increased cancer risk.

Cancer and plastics
- To avoid releasing dioxins from plastics, abstain from using plastic containers and plastic wrap when using the microwave, and do not put plastic water bottles in the freezer.

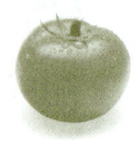

Caffeine and cancer

- Bladder cancer + ☕ ☕ = 2 x risk
- Pancreatic cancer 🚫☕ = 0
- Colon cancer + ☕ ☕ = 1.66 x risk

Increased mortality rates of meat users

(using meat 4+ days a week)
All causes – 33%
Breast cancer – 28%
Ovarian cancer – 66%
Prostate cancer – 51%

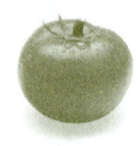

Cancer and red meats

- Having 1 ½ servings of red meat daily almost doubled the risk of hormone receptor-positive breast cancer compared with three or less such meals weekly.
- Older, postmenopausal women who ate 2 oz/57gms of red meat daily had a 56% increased risk of breast cancer compared with those who do not eat red meats.

More on red meat!
- People eating red and processed meats such as hamburgers and luncheon meat have the highest risk for colon and rectal cancers.

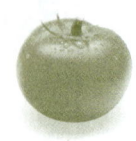

Oh, sugar!

- A sugar called *N-glycolylneuramic acid* (Neu5Gc), and not produced in the human body, is found in high levels in beef, lamb and pork.
- The sugar is viewed by the body as an invader triggering the immune system to a response that can lead to cancer over time.

University of California in San Diego

Associations between selected dietary components and cancer

Site of cancer	Fat	Body weight	Fibre	Fruits & Vegetables	Alcohol	Smoked, salted and pickled foods
Lung				−		
Breast	+	+			+/−	
Colon	++		−	−		
Prostate	++					
Bladder				−		
Rectum	+			−	+	
Endometrium		++				
Oral cavity			−	−	+x	
Stomach				−		++
Cervix				−		
Oesophagus				−	++x	+

+ = Positive association: increased intake associated with increased cancer.
− = Negative association: increased intake associated with decreased cancer.
x = Synergistic with smoking.

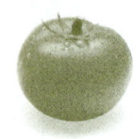

Food and cancer

- People may be protected from cancers associated with the digestive system through eating foods with fibre, folic acid, polyunsaturated fatty acids, flavonoids, and gut fermentation products such as butyrate.
- *Cox-2* enzymes (which enable faulty cells to survive) are suppressed by *quercetin* found in apples and onions.

Another dark side to cancer!

- Dark-colour fruits containing *anthocyanins* can slow the growth of colon cancer by killing up to 20% of the cancerous cells.
- Fruits and vegetables include: bilberries, chokeberries, black carrots, purple corn and radishes.

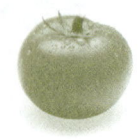

Food sources of known cancer-fighting phytochemicals

Allyl sulphides – chives, garlic, leeks, onions
Caffeic acid – fruits
Carotenoids – green leafy vegetables, red fruits, yellow-orange fruits and vegetables
Curcumins – ginger, turmeric
Dithiolthiones – broccoli
Ellagic acid – grapes, nuts, raspberries, strawberries
Indoles and isothiocyanates – cabbage, cauliflower, broccoli
Isoflavones and saponins – legumes, soybeans, tofu
Lignans – flaxseed, soybeans

Limonene – cardamom, caraway, celery seed, citrus fruits, coriander, dill, fennel
Peitc – watercress
Phenolic acids – berries, grapes, nuts, whole grains
Phytic acid – grains
Protease inhibitors – legumes, soybeans
Resveratrol – red grapes, red-skinned fruits and vegetables
Sinigrin – Brussels sprouts
Sulphoraphane – broccoli

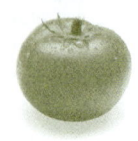

Terpenoids also known to inhibit tumours

Alpha-pinene – caraway, coriander, fennel
Carvone – caraway, dill, spearmint
Geranoil – citrus fruits, coriander, lemongrass, melissa, mint
Menthol – peppermint
Perillyl alcohol – cherries, spearmint
Terpenes – cherries, citrus fruits, herbs

Dietary recommendations

1. Reduce fat intake to 20-30% or less of daily food intake.

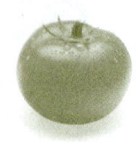

Fat and cancer

- Those women who ate the most fat had an 11% higher incidence of breast cancer than those who ate the least.
- Those with the highest fat intake were also much more likely to have been having hormone replacement therapy (which has been linked separately to breast cancer).

Olive oil

... Javier Menendez ... and his team have shown that oleic acid, the major fatty acid component of olive oil, blocks the production of a protein that boosts the growth of breast cancer cells.
Philip Cohen

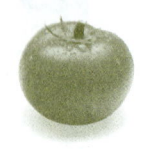

2. Eat more fruits, especially of the vitamin C type.

Vitamin C and cancer growth

- Using high-dose injections of vitamin C may be effective in slowing tumour growth as oral vitamin C is absorbed only in fixed amounts by the digestive system.

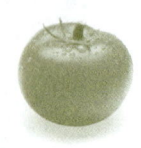

3. Eat more vegetables (especially cruciferous vegetables such as broccoli and cabbage) which are high in vitamin A content.

The sauce of it!
Organic varieties of tomato ketchup contain three times as much of a cancer-fighting chemical called lycopene as non-organic brands. . . . The chemical has been shown to help protect against breast, pancreatic, prostate and intestinal cancer, especially when eaten with fatty foods.
Betty Ishida, Mary Chapman

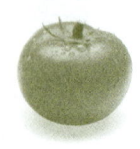

4. Eat more whole grains.

5. Eat less salt-cured, salt-pickled, and smoked foods.

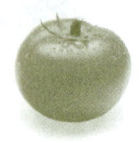

6.
Avoid alcohol.

Alcohol and cancer
- Alcohol increases the body's production of *vascular endothelial growth factor* (VEGF).
- Two alcoholic drinks a day can cause tumour growth (in terms of rapidity and size).

Professors Wei Tan and Jian-Wei Gu, University of Mississippi 2006

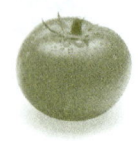

Alcohol

- Oesophageal cancer 17 times higher in alcoholics.
- Mouth and pharyngeal cancer 2-3 times higher in drinkers.
- Laryngeal cancer – higher risk if the person smokes and drinks.
- Liver cancer higher in alcoholic cirrhosis.
- Alcohol = 3% of cancer deaths.

Exercising caution

Change in bowel or bladder habits
A sore that does not heal
Unusual bleeding or discharge
Thickening or lump in the breasts (women and men) or elsewhere
Indigestion or difficulty in swallowing
Obvious change in a wart or mole
Nagging cough or hoarseness that hangs on
American Cancer Society

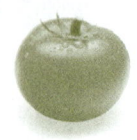

Male cancer mortality ratios
(Smokers vs non-smokers)

Cancer	Age 45-64	Age 65-79
Bladder	2.00	2.96
Kidney	1.42	1.57
Larynx	6.09	8.99
Leukaemia	1.40	1.68
Liver, etc	2.84	1.34
Lung	7.84	11.59
Lymphoma	1.38	0.80
Mouth, pharynx	9.90	2.93
Oesophagus	4.17	1.74
Pancreas	2.69	2.17
Stomach	1.42	1.26
Total cancer	**2.14**	**1.76**

Testicular
self-examination
- When warm and relaxed (best in the bath).
- Feel for the firm, smooth, oval-shaped but irregular-sized organs.
- Examine the softer side and upper portion (the *epididymis* and cord-like tubes).
- If there are any odd lumps or swellings consult your GP.

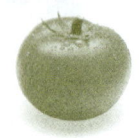

A summary of risk reduction

- Keep your body's resistance high.
- Avoid tobacco and alcohol.
- Keep your weight down.
- Eat foods in as natural a state as possible.
- Avoid a high-animal-fat diet.
- Eat lots of vitamin C fruits.

- Have more vegetables rich in vitamin A.
- Use whole grains and get adequate fibre.
- Protect your skin from too much sun exposure.
- Women should get *PAP* smears done regularly.
- Do breast self-examinations monthly (men too).
- Know the **CAUTION** signs and see your doctor immediately if any occur.

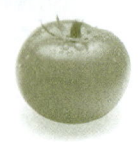

> On a worldwide scale the differences in incidence that have been observed encourage the belief that all the common types of cancer are largely avoidable, in the sense that it should be possible to reduce the risk of developing each type by at least a half and often by 80% or more.
> *Professor Sir Richard Doll*

These three top cancer fighters can help you and your family reduce cancer risks

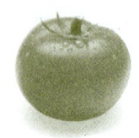

Choose life

Choose life – only that and always, and at whatever risk. To let life leak out, to let it wear away by the mere passage of time, to withhold giving it and spreading it, is to choose nothing.
Sister Helen Kelley